Volume VII

No. 72

March, 1969

Crisis in Psychiatric Hospitalization

*Formulated by
the Committee on Therapeutic Care*

Group for the Advancement of Psychiatry

Additional copies of this GAP Publication No. 72 are available at the following prices: 1-9 copies, $1.00 each; 10-24 copies, list less 15 per cent; 25-99 copies, list less 20 per cent; 100-499 copies, list less 30 per cent.

Upon request the Publications Office of the Group for the Advancement of Psychiatry will provide a complete listing of GAP titles currently in print, quantity prices, and information on subscriptions assuring the receipt of new publications as they are released.

Orders amounting to less than $3.00 must be accompanied by remittance. All prices are subject to change without notice.

Please send your order and remittance to: Publications Office, Group for the Advancement of Psychiatry, 419 Park Avenue South, New York, New York 10016.

Standard Book Number 87318-101-8

Library of Congress Catalog Card Number 62-2872

Printed in the United States of America

Table of Contents

This is the third in a series of publications comprising Volume VII. For a list of other GAP publications on topics related to this subject, please see page 91.

STATEMENT OF PURPOSE

THE GROUP FOR THE ADVANCEMENT OF PSYCHIATRY has a membership of approximately 195 psychiatrists, organized in the form of a number of working committees that direct their efforts toward the study of various aspects of psychiatry and toward the application of this knowledge to the fields of mental health and human relations.

Collaboration with specialists in other disciplines has been and is one of GAP's working principles. Since the formation of GAP in 1946 its members have worked closely with such other specialists as anthropologists, biologists, economists, statisticians, educators, lawyers, nurses, psychologists, sociologists, social workers, and experts in mass communication, philosophy, and semantics. GAP envisages a continuing program of work according to the following aims:

1. To collect and appraise significant data in the field of psychiatry, mental health, and human relations;
2. To re-evaluate old concepts and to develop and test new ones;
3. To apply the knowledge thus obtained for the promotion of mental health and good human relations.

GAP is an independent group and its reports represent the composite findings and opinions of its members only, guided by its many consultants.

CRISIS IN PSYCHIATRIC HOSPITALIZATION *was formulated by the Committee on Therapeutic Care.* The members of this committee as well as all other committees are listed below.*

---

* The present roster of the Committee on Therapeutic Care includes those members who wrote the report. Dr. Marvin L. Adland was an active member of the committee during the time the report was written.

A number of colleagues have assisted us. We wish to acknowledge and express our thanks for their help. Dr. John Cumming and Dr. Sanbourne J. Bockoven aided us in the early development of the theme of the report. Dr. Daniel J. Levinson and Dr. Martin C. Sampson served as consultants to the committee during the writing of the report. Three Sol Ginsburg Group for the Advancement of Psychiatry Fellows have contributed to the committee's work: Dr. Lloyd C. Elam, Dr. Herzl R. Spiro, and Dr. Cullen R. Schwemer.

We acknowledge with gratitude the financial assistance from Wallace Pharmaceuticals, Division of Carter-Wallace, Inc.

Committee on Therapeutic Care
Benjamin Simon, Boston, Chr.
Ian L. W. Clancey, Ottawa
Thomas E. Curtis, Chapel Hill
Robert W. Gibson, Towson, Md.
Harold A. Greenberg, Bethesda
Henry U. Grunebaum, Boston
Bernard H. Hall, Topeka
Lester H. Rudy, Chicago
Melvin Sabshin, Chicago
Robert E. Switzer, Topeka

Committee on Adolescence
Joseph D. Noshpitz, Washington, D.C.,
    Chr.
Warren J. Gadpaille, Denver
Mary O'Neil Hawkins, New York
Charles A. Malone, Philadelphia
Silvio J. Onesti, Jr., Boston
Vivian Rakoff, Montreal
Calvin F. Settlage, Ardmore, Pa.
Sidney L. Werkman, Washington, D.C.

Committee on Aging
Jack Weinberg, Chicago, Chr.
Robert N. Butler, Washington, D.C.
Alvin I. Goldfarb, New York
Lawrence F. Greenleigh, Los Angeles
Maurice E. Linden, Philadelphia
Prescott W. Thompson, Topeka
Montague Ullman, Brooklyn

Committee on Child Psychiatry
E. James Anthony, St. Louis, Chr.
Suzanne T. van Amerongen, Boston
James M. Bell, New Canaan, N.Y.
H. Donald Dunton, New York
Joseph M. Green, Tucson, Ariz.
John F. Kenward, Chicago
William S. Langford, New York
John F. McDermott, Jr., Ann Arbor
Dane G. Prugh, Denver
Exie E. Welsch, New York
Virginia N. Wilking, New York

Committee on College Student
Harrison P. Eddy, New York, Chr.
Robert L. Arnstein, New Haven
Alfred Flarsheim, Chicago
Alan Frank, Albuquerque, N.M.
Malkah Tolpin Notman, Brookline, Mass.
Kent E. Robinson, Towson, Md.
Earle Silber, Washington, D.C.
Benson R. Snyder, Cambridge
Tom G. Stauffer, Scarsdale, N.Y.
J. B. Wheelwright, San Francisco

Committee on the Family
Israel Zwerling, New York, Chr.
Ivan Boszormenyi-Nagy, Philadelphia
L. Murray Bowen, Chevy Chase
David Mendell, Houston
Norman L. Paul, Cambridge
Joseph Satten, Topeka
Kurt O. Schlesinger, San Francisco
John P. Spiegel, Waltham, Mass.
Lyman C. Wynne, Bethesda

Committee on
Governmental Agencies
Harold Rosen, Baltimore, Chr.
Calvin S. Drayer, Philadelphia
Edward O. Harper, Cleveland
John E. Nardini, Washington, D.C.
Donald B. Peterson, Fulton, Mo.
Robert L. Williams, Gainesville, Fla.

Committee on
International Relations
Robert L. Leopold, Philadelphia, Chr.
Francis F. Barnes, Chevy Chase
Eugene Brody, Baltimore
William D. Davidson, Washington, D.C.
Joseph T. English, Washington, D.C.
Louis C. English, Pomona, N.Y.
Frank Fremont-Smith, Massapequa, N.Y.
John A. P. Millet, New York
Alain J. Sanseigne, New York
Bertram Schaffner, New York
Mottram P. Torre, New Orleans
Byrant M. Wedge, West Medford, Mass.

COMMITTEE ON MEDICAL EDUCATION
David R. Hawkins, Charlottesville, Chr.
Hugh T. Carmichael, Washington, D.C.
Robert S. Daniels, Chicago
Raymond Feldman, Boulder, Colo.
Saul I. Harrison, Ann Arbor
Harold I. Lief, Philadelphia
John E. Mack, Boston
Herbert C. Modlin, Topeka
William L. Peltz, Philadelphia
David S. Sanders, Los Angeles
Robert A. Senescu, Albuquerque, N.M.
Roy M. Whitman, Cincinnati

COMMITTEE ON
MENTAL HEALTH SERVICES
Lucy D. Ozarin, Bethesda, Chr.
Morris E. Chafetz, Boston
Merrill Eaton, Omaha
James B. Funkhouser, Richmond, Va.
Robert S. Garber, Belle Mead, N.J.
Ernest W. Klatte, Talmage, Calif.
Alan I. Levenson, Chevy Chase
W. Walter Menninger, Topeka
Lee G. Sewall, N. Little Rock, Ark.
Jack A. Wolford, Pittsburgh

COMMITTEE ON
MENTAL RETARDATION
Henry H. Work, Los Angeles, Chr.
Howard V. Bair, Parsons, Kans.
Peter W. Bowman, Pownal, Me.
Stuart M. Finch, Ann Arbor
Leo Madow, Philadelphia
Irving Philips, San Francisco
George Tarjan, Los Angeles
Warren T. Vaughan, Jr., San Mateo
Thomas G. Webster, Bethesda

COMMITTEE ON
PREVENTIVE PSYCHIATRY
Stephen Fleck, New Haven, Chr.
Gerald Caplan, Boston
Jules V. Coleman, New Haven
Leonard J. Duhl, Berkeley

Albert J. Glass, Oklahoma City
Benjamin Jeffries, Harper Woods, Mich.
E. James Lieberman, Washington, D.C.,
Mary E. Mercer, Nyack, N.Y.
Harris B. Peck, Bronx, N.Y.
Marvin E. Perkins, New York
Harold M. Visotsky, Chicago
Stanley F. Yolles, Bethesda

COMMITTEE ON
PSYCHIATRY AND LAW
Zigmond M. Lebensohn, Washington,
  D.C., Chr.
Edward T. Auer, St. Louis
John Donnelly, Hartford
Jay Katz, New Haven
Carl P. Malmquist, Minneapolis
Seymour Pollack, Los Angeles
Alan A. Stone, Cambridge
Gene L. Usdin, New Orleans
Andrew S. Watson, Ann Arbor

COMMITTEE ON
PSYCHIATRY AND RELIGION
Earl A. Loomis, Jr., New York, Chr.
Arthur J. Deikman, Denver
Sidney S. Furst, New York
Stanley A. Leavy, New Haven
Albert J. Lubin, Woodside, Calif.
Mortimer Ostow, New York

COMMITTEE ON
PSYCHIATRY AND SOCIAL WORK
C. Knight Aldrich, Chicago
Maurice R. Friend, New York
John A. MacLeod, Cincinnati
John C. Nemiah, Boston
Eleanor A. Steele, Denver

COMMITTEE ON
PSYCHIATRY IN INDUSTRY
Harry H. Wagenheim, Philadelphia, Chr.
Spencer Bayles, Houston
Thomas L. Brannick, Rochester, Minn.
Herbert L. Klemme, Topeka
Jeptha R. MacFarlane, Westbury, N.Y.

Alan A. McLean, New York
Kenneth J. Munden, Memphis
Clarence J. Rowe, St. Paul
Graham C. Taylor, Montreal

COMMITTEE ON PSYCHOPATHOLOGY
Albert J. Silverman, New Brunswick, N.J., Chr.
Wagner H. Bridger, New York
Neil R. Burch, Houston
Sanford I. Cohen, New Orleans
James H. Ewing, Wallingford, Pa.
Daniel X. Freedman, Chicago
Milton Greenblatt, Boston
Paul E. Huston, Iowa City
P. Herbert Leiderman, Palo Alto, Calif.
Jack H. Mendelson, Chevy Chase
George E. Ruff, Philadelphia
Charles Shagass, Philadelphia
Marvin Stein, Brooklyn
George E. Vaillant, Boston

COMMITTEE ON PUBLIC EDUCATION
Peter A. Martin, Detroit, Chr.
Leo H. Bartemeier, Baltimore
H. Waldo Bird, El Paso, Texas
Lloyd C. Elam, Nashville
Dana L. Farnsworth, Cambridge
John P. Lambert, Katonah, N.Y.
Mildred Mitchell-Bateman, Charleston
Mabel Ross, Boston
Julius Schreiber, Washington, D.C.
Kent A. Zimmerman, Berkeley

COMMITTEE ON RESEARCH
Morris A. Lipton, Chapel Hill, Chr.
Stanley Eldred, Belmont, Mass.
Louis A. Gottschalk, Irvine, Calif.
Sheppard G. Kellam, Chicago
Gerald L. Klerman, New Haven
Ralph R. Notman, Brookline, Mass.
Franz K. Reichsman, Brooklyn
Richard E. Renneker, Los Angeles
Alfred H. Stanton, Boston

COMMITTEE ON SOCIAL ISSUES
Perry Ottenberg, Philadelphia, Chr.
Viola W. Bernard, New York

Robert Coles, Cambridge
Lester Grinspoon, Boston
Joel S. Handler, Chicago
Judd Marmor, Los Angeles
Roy W. Menninger, Topeka
Arthur A. Miller, Chicago
Peter B. Neubauer, New York
Charles A. Pinderhughes, Boston
Kendon W. Smith, Piermont, N.Y.

COMMITTEE ON THERAPY
Peter H. Knapp, Boston, Chr.
Henry W. Brosin, Pittsburgh
Eugene Meyer, Baltimore
William C. Offenkrantz, Chicago
Lewis L. Robbins, Glen Oaks, N.Y.
Albert E. Scheflen, Bronx, N.Y.
Harley C. Shands, New York
Lucia E. Tower, Chicago

CONTRIBUTING MEMBERS
Marvin L. Adland, Chevy Chase
Carlos C. Alden, Jr., Williamsville
William H. Anderson, Lansing, Mich.
Kenneth E. Appel, Philadelphia
M. Royden C. Astley, Pittsburgh
Charlotte Babcock, Pittsburgh
Grace Baker, New York
Benjamin H. Balser, New York
Bernard Bandler, Boston
Walter E. Barton, Washington, D.C.
Anna R. Benjamin, Chicago
Ivan C. Berlien, Coral Gables, Fla.
Sidney Berman, Washington, D.C.
Grete L. Bibring, Cambridge
Edward G. Billings, Denver
Carl A. L. Binger, Cambridge
Wilfred Bloomberg, Hartford
C. H. Hardin Branch, Salt Lake City
Matthew Brody, Brooklyn
Ewald W. Busse, Durham
Dale C. Cameron, Geneva
Norman Cameron, New Haven
Harvey H. Corman, New York
Frank J. Curran, New York
Bernard L. Diamond, Berkeley
Franklin G. Ebaugh, Denver

Joel Elkes, Baltimore
O. Spurgeon English, Narbeth, Pa.
Jack R. Ewalt, Boston
Lawrence Z. Freedman, Stanford
Moses M. Frohlich, Ann Arbor
Daniel H. Funkenstein, Boston
Maurice H. Greenhill, Scarsdale, N.Y.
John H. Greist, Indianapolis
Roy R. Grinker, Chicago
Ernest M. Gruenberg, New York
Herbert I. Harris, Cambridge
J. Cotter Hirschberg, Topeka
Edward J. Hornick, New York
Edward William Howell, Ann Arbor
Joseph Hughes, Philadelphia
Portia Bell Hume, Berkeley
Robert W. Hyde, Waterbury, Vt.
Lucie Jessner, Washington, D.C.
Irene M. Josselyn, Phoenix
Marion E. Kenworthy, New York
Edward J. Kollar, Tucson, Ariz.
Othilda Krug, Cincinnati
Lawrence S. Kubie, Sparks, Md.
Paul V. Lemkau, Baltimore
Maurice Levine, Cincinnati
David M. Levy, New York
Robert J. Lifton, Woodbridge, Conn.
Erich Lindemann, Palo Alto, Calif.
Reginald S. Lourie, Washington, D.C.
Alfred O. Ludwig, Boston
Sydney G. Margolin, Denver
Helen V. McLean, Chicago
Karl Menninger, Topeka
James G. Miller, Cleveland
Angel N. Miranda, Hato Pey, P.R.
Rudolph G. Novick, Lincolnwood, Ill.
Francis J. O'Neill, Central Islip, N.J.
Humphry F. Osmond, Princeton, N.J.
Eveoleen N. Rexford, Cambridge
Milton Rosenbaum, New York
Mathew Ross, Chestnut Hill, Mass.
W. Donald Ross, Cincinnati
Elvin M. Semrad, Boston
Edward Stainbrook, Los Angeles
Brandt F. Steele, Denver
Rutherford B. Stevens, New York
Lloyd J. Thompson, Chapel Hill

Harvey J. Tompkins, New York
Arthur F. Valenstein, Cambridge
Helen Stochen Wagenheim, Philadelphia
Raymond W. Waggoner, Ann Arbor
Robert S. Wallerstein, San Francisco
Edward M. Weinshel, San Francisco
Cecil L. Wittson, Omaha
David Wright, Providence

LIFE MEMBERS

S. Spafford Ackerly, Louisville
John R. Rees, London, England
Bruce Robinson, Culver, Ind.
Francis H. Sleeper, Augusta, Me.

OFFICERS

President
Herbert C. Modlin
Box 829, Topeka, Kans. 66601

Vice President
John Donnelly
200 Retreat Avenue
Hartford, Conn. 06102

Secretary-Treasurer
Malcolm J. Farrell
Box C, Waverley, Mass. 02178

Asst. Secretary-Treasurer
Paul E. Huston
500 Newton Road
Iowa City, Iowa 52241

PUBLICATIONS BOARD

Chairman
Milton Greenblatt
15 Ashburton Place
Boston, Mass. 02108

Maurice R. Friend
Louis A. Gottschalk
Bernard M. Hall
John C. Nemiah
Perry Ottenberg
Henry H. Work

INTRODUCTION

This report is a protest against a current bandwagon movement exemplified by such slogans as: *Keep patients out of psychiatric hospitals as much as you can; Use the psychiatric ward of a general hospital instead of a mental hospital; The only good psychiatry is treatment in the community.* This report emphasizes the vital role of the psychiatric hospital in a continuum of comprehensive psychiatric treatment.

Years of study, treatment, and research in psychiatric hospitals have provided insights into the spectrum of forces that influence mental health and mental illness. Concurrent studies of the psychodynamics of personality development and family interaction have resulted in a rich clinical awareness of the psychological strengths and weaknesses that exist within the individual, his family, and his community. These studies have generated a new hope for the mentally ill. An expanding array of therapeutic techniques and therapeutic settings has resulted. There is an increasing emphasis on the early recognition of emotional problems and on treatment of the patient as close to his family-community setting as possible. Many disabling symptoms of mental illness can now be alleviated by the use of new pharmacological agents developed through biochemical research.

A vast complex of therapeutic settings has been developed— community mental health centers, psychiatric units in general hospitals, day, night, and weekend hospitals, halfway houses, and sheltered workshops. All of these new treatment approaches are designed to interrupt emotional illness early and to treat the patient as close to his home as possible. We believe that such treatment innovations have great merit, but we are concerned that their use has evolved into movements to abolish the psychiatric hospital. We wish to identify and assess the issues involved. The basic clinical question is: *What diagnostic and treatment services are required to facilitate the patient's recovery?*

The psychiatric hospital is an integral and necessary component of the therapeutic continuum. It need not be a social anachronism. It should be a responsible institution, sensitive to social change and dedicated to the care of the sick. When properly structured, efficiently administered, and intelligently staffed, the psychiatric hospital provides a singularly important part of comprehensive psychiatric care.

The current crisis about the use of the psychiatric hospital reflects forces that are unprecedented in the history of therapeutic care for the mentally ill. During the 1960's in the United States, a distinct trend has changed into an active movement that now challenges the functional utility of psychiatric hospitals. The slogans that we have enumerated above state the challenge quite explicitly. Those who say "keep the patient out of the hospital at all cost" are, in effect, denying the positive aspects of therapeutic care that psychiatric hospitals have provided and continue to provide.

The effect of such attitudes can be seen in the Medicare-Medicaid legislation. The first version (H.R. 1, King-Anderson) contained a simple clause excluding treatment in any institution that was primarily for the care of the mentally ill. No limitation whatsoever was made on benefits for treatment in a psychiatric unit of a general hospital.

Many psychiatrists, recognizing the important role of the psychiatric hospital, protested and were vigorously supported by the American Psychiatric Association and the National Association for Mental Health. Through their efforts the *Medicare* benefits were expanded to include treatment in a psychiatric hospital, but with significant restrictions. The *Medicaid* benefits for persons under 65 were not changed and still exclude treatment in a psychiatric hospital. And yet, no special restrictions whatsoever are applied to the psychiatric unit of a general hospital. These actions by the Congress clearly reflect the influence the campaign against psychiatric hospitals has had on federal officials. It is a striking illustration of the damaging impact the movement against psychiatric hospitals has had on the care of the psychiatric patient.

What is unprecedented in the current crisis is the undeniable fact that those who question the value of psychiatric hospitals today are motivated by humane and progressive concepts. They genuinely *care* about mentally ill people. They wish to provide adequate care for *all* members of a community who are psychiatrically ill, regardless of their economic and social status. Furthermore, they wish to maintain the intactness of the patient's family and work status by treating him as close to home as is possible. In attempting to improve psychiatric care, however, they maintain that a psychiatric hospital can only be a barren repository for people who cannot obtain adequate care elsewhere. To keep them out of such dreary circumstances at all costs is a significant and noble effort, but the overzealous application of this attempt may lead to a variety of unintended consequences. Indeed, there is the distinct possibility that such an overzealous application may unintentionally induce massive retrogressive changes in our psychiatric hospitals.

Ironically enough, those who advocate the anti-hospital slogans today on humanist grounds may find themselves aligned with current and historical forces whose anti-mental health bias has been based on an antihumanist position. For hundreds of years struggles have taken place between those who wished to provide humane treatment for the mentally ill and those who opposed it or were apathetic to such efforts under one guise or another.

The libertarian values of the French and American revolutions were reflected in the actions of Pinel and the American advocates of Moral Treatment. Those values achieved ascendency in the first half of the 19th century. In the latter half of that century, they were eroded in the United States by those who preached therapeutic pessimism, those prejudiced against the poor, and those who thought that such humanitarian values were too costly.

It was not until after World War II that a determined and persistent national effort was generated to introduce therapeutic principles into the large public mental hospitals. Despite this effort, many of these hospitals remain distressingly inadequate. In fact, some of the drive that led to the development of community treatment resulted from the feeling that these hospitals could not be changed. During the 1950's, significant improvement began to be apparent. Psychiatric hospitals began to be an exciting setting in which to innovate therapeutic principles and practices. Careers in hospital psychiatry began to become attractive to bright young psychiatric residents who could envisage a satisfying professional career in psychiatric hospital work. Research efforts in and about psychiatric hospitals achieved a peak with a variety of imaginative hypotheses. The stigma of mental hospitalization began to be reduced and the boundary between the hospital and the community became increasingly permeable. The hospital psychiatry of the 1950's gave force and sustenance to the community psychiatry of the 1960's.

It would be ironic indeed if the increased permeability from hospital to community helped to pave the way toward dissolution of the psychiatric hospital. Those who state that treatment in the community without recourse to hospitalization is the only good psychiatry may contribute to such a dissolution, but what will also dissolve will be all of the progressive advances made in hospital psychiatry during the past two decades. The new slogans will not in actuality lead to the tearing down of all psychiatric hospitals. Rather they will lead to our psychiatric hospitals again becoming repositories for those patients who have failed to respond to alternative forms of therapy. A new, more insidious period of custodial care may ensue, and once again the mentally ill will be abandoned and isolated.

In this report we wish to emphasize the positive aspects of psychiatric hospitalization that have existed for centuries, even if they were less in evidence during periods of neglect and isolation. The need for psychological retreats for those under stress has been apparent since antiquity, but the retreat function of the hospital has been complemented during the last 50 years by active therapeutic modalities that are best employed in the psychiatric hospital. We shall demonstrate the advantages of the applications of these modalities by discussing admission, treatment, and discharge from the psychiatric hospital. We shall describe some of the frequent issues that arise and that demand clinical consideration during the various phases of therapeutic care in order to illustrate the positive functions of the hospital.

1

INDICATIONS FOR HOSPITALIZATION

The reasons for admission to a general medical or to a psychiatric hospital are similar. From the standpoint of the patient, hospital admission is recommended when (a) skilled clinical observation is needed for diagnostic clarification; and (b) special medical, nursing, and rehabilitative treatment is required. From the standpoint of society the hospital is required (a) to protect society from the effects of the patient's illness (self-destructive or homicidal behavior); and (b) to protect a family and society from the exhaustion of its resources by the disorganizing impact of the patient's acute or chronic illness.

These are positive reasons for hospital care. We do not believe that optimal hospital use requires that all other resources be exhausted. This represents hospital care by default. Unfortunately, probably more than half of the admissions to psychiatric hospitals result from "default"; "nothing else worked, so we brought him here," as many families say. Glaring indications for psychiatric hospitalization were apparent much earlier and were not recognized.

There are circumstances through which the progression of illness can be interrupted without hospital care. (For example: by removing the person from the conflict-provoking situations; by relieving the patient of social responsibilities; by the use of psychopharmacologic agents or electroconvulsive treatment; or by establishing a working relationship with a psychotherapist). These techniques may provide relief from pressure, may provide insight, and may lead either to recovery of old adequate psychological defenses or to new and better ones. For some patients this may be appropriate. For others it would simply prolong a less-than-optimal adjustment. For still others, it could cause a disastrous postponement of needed therapeutic intervention by not hospitalizing the patient.

What then does the psychiatric hospital provide that makes it particularly effective in helping the troubled person?

In its diagnostic and therapeutic functions the hospital provides a concentration of skilled professionals competent to deal with the patient, family, and community in a consistent manner. In this setting the gathering of information and the therapeutic use of information are inseparable and part of the total daily hospital life. Diagnostic and treatment modalities to meet the medical and social needs may be found elsewhere but seldom in such complete and accessible combination. Although the diagnostic and therapeutic procedures are intimately interwoven, for purposes of clarity of exposition we will for the moment deal with them separately.

Hospitalization for diagnostic purposes includes:

1. Extended observation of the patient's behavior and his mode of relating to others.
2. Clarification of discrepancies between the patient's complaints and the reports of those with whom he lives.
3. Determination of how much of the picture presented by the patient is due to a situational conflict and how much to an intrapsychic conflict.

Hospitalization for treatment is indicated when:

1. Supportive measures have been unsuccessful in halting or reversing the regressive process.
2. The magnitude of regressive, depressive, or aggressive behavior is no longer tolerable to the patient and/or society.
3. The management of special treatments, somatic procedures, and psychopharmacologic drugs requires continuous observation.

4. A controlled environment is essential for the use of psychotherapy.
5. Medications or drugs on which the patient has become dependent must be withdrawn.

An individual's need for hospitalization, therefore, involves an examination of his personal problems and an assessment of his personal and the community resources. If the totality of resources, including alternative management procedures, is inadequate, hospitalization may be clearly indicated. The child who is performing poorly in school, home, and social relationships with his peers because of conflict may be maintained outside a hospital when supports such as family participation, school counseling, and clinic or private outpatient care are available. On the other hand, it is seldom possible to provide the external supports required to maintain a severely disturbed child out of a hospital. The emphasis should be on providing a total treatment approach that has the most significant rewards in developing a healthy personality or preventing destructive regression, rather than mere avoidance of hospitalization.

Case Example

A 10-year-old boy had been unable to swallow solid foods for six months. His mother reported that he seemed to be afraid that something was lodged in his throat that made the swallowing of solids impossible. He repeatedly asked his mother to look at his throat. The patient had limited his diet to fruit juices mixed with raw eggs and sugar, consomme, milk, and ice cream.

The boy's relationship with his mother was observed to be a very dependent one. He was possessive and demanding of her. He was frail, spoke softly, and frequently shut his eyes in tic-like spasms. He was reticent to talk about his experiences, relationships, and activities. His behavior fluctuated from a logical, reality-bound approach to fluid, fantastic productions.

To adequately treat this young patient required psychiatric hospitalization that included individual psychotherapy, special education, and active casework with the parents.

When an individual poses a persistent threat to the family, community, or himself, hospitalization is clearly indicated as an emergency measure. Admission does not await a complete examination of the patient. Few would disagree that psychiatric hospitalization is the treatment of choice for an individual who is actively suicidal.

Although acutely depressed individuals can be managed in alternate settings, hospitalization is usually preferable. It is only in the hospital that total observation or evaluation of the individual is possible, as well as an assessment of the meaningful interactions of the patient, staff, and other patients.

Psychiatric hospitalization may also be an emergency recourse when an individual has become threatening toward others because of paranoid projections, delusions, and breakdown of control. It is also often required on an emergency basis in states of acute anxiety or panic that may be on a toxic or psychological basis. The panic state requires immediate withdrawal from current environment. Frequently, episodes of acute decompensation observed in senile and arteriosclerotic patients respond well to prompt and short-term hospital care.

In still other instances the need for hospitalization is less apparent. Although a patient's maladaptive psychological state may not be extreme, his illness may have caused severe family disequilibrium. If the resources of the family are strained to the limit, hospitalization may be indicated to enable the family to restore its balance.

Case Example

A 23-year-old student on insulin therapy for diabetes became almost completely preoccupied with the care and cleaning of his syringes, the time of injections, and the details of his treatment. His severely compulsive efforts to order his world made life unusually difficult for his family and associates. He needed the hospital to spare the family, to relieve him of responsibility, and to be helped in understanding his anxiety and his behavior.

Occasionally the individual who is hospitalized may not be the sickest member of the family, but his absence from the home may help integrate the others and have a more profound therapeutic effect than if he were in individual treatment. A disruptive member of the family may, of course, be separated by means other than hospitalization, such as visits to another city, general hospital admission, or halfway-house care. In evaluating the need for hospitalization, these alternatives may be balanced against the particular problems involved.

Case Example

> A 25-year-old man was admitted to a psychiatric hospital because of alarming episodes of "wild" activity and self-mutilation at home. Later the same year, his 27-year-old sister was also admitted in a state of hallucinatory and paranoid fearfulness. Since their late teens, both patients had had numerous psychotic episodes that characteristically quickly remitted and then rapidly recurred.
>
> A diagnostic assessment of the entire family revealed that the illness in the children was a reflection of serious disequilibrium within the family. The hospital staff concluded that no change in the course of the illness could be expected until the children received long-term treatment in a hospital setting and the parents were provided with psychiatric help. Further, it was felt that the total administrative support of the hospital and the therapeutic skills of the staff had to be committed over an extended time to accomplish the treatment task. The family-hospital effort subsequently continued over a period of four years.

There are a variety of long-standing psychological difficulties that are not emergencies but are best handled by hospitalization. One such commonly overlooked situation involves the need to permit regression within the sanctuary of the psychiatric hospital. In contrast to the home where uncontrolled regressive behavior may be severely disruptive to the family, the hospital can allow the patient to undergo "controlled" regression in order to reconstitute defenses in a healthier fashion.

Case Example

A 47-year-old executive was admitted to a psychiatric hospital because of depression manifested by feelings of rejection, despair, constricting interests in work and family situations, and some feelings of guilt over his having sacrificed family relations in his drive for business success. When the youngest child left home for college, the patient's symptoms became exaggerated and he was hospitalized. The "loss" of the child had awakened anger and guilt. It also awakened his awareness that his own needs were not being fully gratified by his business successes and had only accentuated his feelings of loneliness. The optimum treatment for this individual was a controlled regression that could not be handled in any other treatment situation. This patient was removed from the home setting of acute loss and failure. His dependency needs were met, while at the same time he was helped to become aware of his needs, conflicts, and guilt. He gradually left his room on the ward, entered into the patient group, and made a satisfactory recovery.

It may be useful to bring conflicts forcefully into the open so that they may be resolved. The setting of a hospital can simultaneously provide the necessary support to the patient in his dependent needs, while forcing an examination of his conflicts.

Case Example

A 19-year-old girl with manifest aggressivity and hostility toward her divorced mother with whom she was living entered a psychiatric hospital on a court order. The hospital was able to offer the consistent attitudes and controls that this girl had never experienced.

Brief hospitalization is frequently indicated to assess and to adjust drug dosage levels in long-term psychiatric care. With the advent of the tranquilizer and antidepressant drugs, long-term medication has become common, and yet it is often not carefully regulated from the viewpoint of dosage and untoward reactions. In certain cases hospitalization is indicated for control or change of medication.

2

ADMISSION TO THE PSYCHIATRIC HOSPITAL

Many patients and their families regard admission to a mental hospital as a declaration of personal failure. Even some mental health professionals share this point of view. This misconception is communicated to patients who are denied this valuable resource. We wish to emphasize that hospitalization is not a defeat; quite the contrary, it should be a positive step toward health.

In some situations a barrier to hospitalization may well be the mutual patient and family reluctance to acknowledge and to disrupt a pattern that, though pathological, satisfied their needs. The threat of loss of familiar people, objects, or a work situation is also perceived as disturbing. To the paranoid patient the external world is dangerous or turbulent, and he denies his own part in the illness in a truculent fashion.

Because of these many doubts and resistances, the admission process should include participation by the patient and the patient's family in assessing the needs for hospitalization. Too often patients and their families expect a magical cure or the enrichment of an individual to a status far beyond that of his previous best adjustment. When this expectation is not fulfilled, the disappointment can lead to a rejection of the patient by his family and a rejection of the hospital and/or family by the patient. Under such circumstances the patient and/or his family may precipitate a premature hospital discharge against medical advice.

While denial of illness is a problem present in all areas of medical care and hospitalization, it is especially common in psychiatric hospitalization and is a significant and complicating factor.

Drugs can be used effectively to lessen aggressive impulses and suffering. But they can also be withheld or reduced when it is in the best interest of the patient. The physical protection of the hospital minimizes the possibility of self-harm from aggressive impulses, loss of sexual control, and abuse of alcohol and/or drugs. In certain instances the hospital affords protection for the community against patients having uncontrollable impulses. External controls offer reassurance to the patient and, through identification with the staff, foster ego growth that helps the patient develop his own inner controls.

Disengagement from a pathological constellation is an important use of hospitalization. An adolescent can be removed from an unduly stressful peer-group situation. A destructive work situation may be relieved. The participants in a sadomasochistic marriage may be temporarily separated. By interrupting such destructive interactions, the hospital offers the patient some relief from the situational factors contributing to his difficulties and supports him in gaining a more rational perspective and new adaptive patterns. He then has a better opportunity to master situations that were formerly stressful.

A *controlled treatment program* for some patients can be carried out only in a hospital setting. Regular appointments with the psychotherapist can be scheduled and maintained. The availability of a supportive staff on a 24-hour-a-day basis permits the therapist to deal with anxiety-provoking material that would be overwhelming in a nonprotected situation. The control of behavior can help the patient stop acting out his impulses so that he can reflect about his drives and understand himself. When indicated, medications can be prescribed with the assurance that they will not be misused. The clinical response of the patient to medication can be continually observed. The patient who has become dependent or even addicted can be withdrawn in physical safety and in a setting of emotional support.

A *total and coordinated approach* can be provided for the individual patient in the hospital. The total life pattern of the patient can be directed and utilized as a part of the treatment program. Work, recreation, and varied activities can be used as part of a rehabilitative and re-educational program for the patient. Individual and group interactions, as well as solitude, are available in the hospital. The hospital provides a life situation that facilitates learning in the broadest sense. The patient can admire and identify with the strength of the hospital staff. He can develop new skills and adaptive patterns. These principles about hospital treatment are illustrated in the following clinical example.

Case Example

A 40-year-old woman was referred to the hospital because her psychotherapist considered her behavior too dangerous and disruptive for outpatient treatment. After two years of psychotherapy her first episodes of overactivity and hyperelation occurred. She drank and spent money excessively and had violent arguments with her husband. As this manic episode subsided, she became depressed and received an antidepressant medication but with little benefit. The marital situation became increasingly strained by the patient's excessive spending and neglect of her home and children. Just prior to admission there was a stormy scene when the patient's husband discovered her in a restaurant with another man. The public scandal was intolerable to the husband, and the psychotherapist concluded that the patient should be hospitalized.

The therapist described the damaging interaction between the patient and her husband as follows: "She expressed hostile, resentful feelings toward men and her husband in particular, like cursing, which she knew he abhorred; by spending more money than he deemed prudent, which she well knew would infuriate him; and by criticizing his family, which invariably enraged him." Although the husband could accept the periods of depression and even dangerous suicidal attempts, he found the patient intolerable during periods of excitement, especially when she created a public disturbance. The patient's difficulties totally disrupted the family. Both children began to manifest disturbances of behavior. Efforts were made to assist the children by placing them in private schools, but during the periods of elation the patient disrupted this arrangement by interfering with the children at the schools.

The patient made several suicidal gestures, some of a dramatic quality and consciously calculated to achieve a reconciliation with her husband. She came perilously close to death in these dramatic attempts. On at least two other occasions, when profoundly depressed, she made serious attempts at self-destruction. She drank excessively and showed no regard for her own safety. She jeopardized the family financial position and created scandals that estranged her from all her friends and family.

The patient's behavior had disrupted any real therapeutic work even though intensive psychotherapy on a five-times-a-week basis was attempted. The therapist described her as follows: "She used all her wiles, and was at times seductive both in her associations and in her dream content. When she found this was not effective in manipulating me, she used her illness in order to maintain her hold on me. When I went on vacation with my family, she swung from being depressed into an excited period. There were numerous telephone calls following me on my trip."

During a nine-month hospitalization it was possible to deal with the specific problems that had interfered with treatment outside the hospital. The patient did not present a diagnostic problem in the sense of formal classification; her symptoms and history were typical of a mood disorder. But hospitalization was needed for a full diagnostic assessment of several crucial points. Were the marital difficulties the cause of the patient's illness, and to what degree did they affect the patient's illness? What role did alcohol and drug abuse have in the symptoms? Could she develop a meaningful relationship? To what extent were suicidal threats an indication of depression and to what extent a manipulative acting out? None of these questions had been adequately answered in the several years of treatment prior to hospitalization.

During the patient's hospitalization there were no actual suicidal attempts though she often talked about injuring herself. Within the hospital sufficient precautions and control could be exercised to prevent this. The patient could no longer dominate the people around her through suicidal threats. The therapist and the hospital staff could proceed in their therapeutic efforts with reasonable security and safety.

Hospitalization interrupted the distressing interactions between the patient, her husband, and her children. This gave the patient some distance and perspective on the situation, as well as sparing the children from the destructive impact. She tried to perpetuate the sadomasochistic relationship with her husband through telephone calls, but as this pattern emerged her communications with him were limited to letters. These letters were shared with the patient's hospital physician and provided an opportunity for effectively demonstrating to the patient that she was not an innocent victim but was in fact extraordinarily provocative and a major contributor to the disturbance in her marriage. The husband's monthly visits took place in the presence of a staff member. Toward the end of each visit there was a discussion with the patient and her husband about what had occurred. In this setting the visits were reasonably controlled and the patient and her husband were, for the first time, able to discuss realistically the problems in their marriage without having the situation deteriorate into a shamble of mutual accusations and retaliations.

Psychotherapy could be carried out more effectively. The patient's resistance to therapy could be controlled. The therapist was able to explore anxiety-provoking material without having treatment disrupted by suicidal threats or acting out. Manipulation of the environment made it possible to reinforce and facilitate the insight gained in individual psychotherapy. Having multiple sources of information the therapist could more effectively assess the patient's role in the interplay between her and the environment.

The patient's pattern of provocative and exhibitionistic behavior continued within the hospital. For example, she talked about being a drug addict and an alcoholic, and described in great detail various sexual exploits. On occasion she grabbed at student nurses in what appeared to be a crude sexual approach, saying how pretty they looked. A nurse's note describes her as follows: ". . . she was loud and demanding. She was wearing a very bright lavender strapless sarong and lying on her bed talking in a high-pitched voice and occasionally screaming for medication for her cramps." She spoke of wanting to burn the hospital down, but in a note the nurse wrote, "I do not believe she is dangerous but somehow likes to attract attention to see if the staff will panic."

The total hospital milieu could be mobilized in treating the patient. There were repeated discussions with the patient about her mode of interaction. This was done by staff and by other patients often in critical confrontations of the patient at the regular meetings held by the staff-patient group. Through participation in formal group therapy the patient was able to gain a more accurate picture of her impact on others. Her spending was controlled, and her efforts to manipulate the hospital physician into authorizing excessive purchases were identified and limited. Her reactions to these limitations were explored with her psychotherapist.

The major emphasis in a modern psychiatric hospital is on flexibility of treatment planning. To achieve this the hospital must have staff members from all the mental health disciplines. It must make provision for 24-hour-a-day care, partial hospitalization (day, night, weekend hospitalization), and outpatient services. The hospital must be large enough to provide many services, yet small enough in its functional units so that the needs of the individual patient can be recognized and met.

Many patients need assistance in maintaining community ties and responsibilities. However, nothing should be done for the patient that he can do for himself. Personal, professional, educational, and family responsibilities should be maintained to the extent that they are helpful to the patient. Patients may continue their work, pursue an education, care for children, and live outside of the hospital for a significant part of the time.

Asylum is for some patients the most valuable function of the hospital. Hospitalization may be a retreat in which the patient can re-marshall his forces. He can be sick and at the same time be accepted, wanted, and appreciated.

The patient may be allowed to regress as far as he needs and for as long as he needs. Where this process is accepted, understood, and permitted to take its course without rejection by the hospital staff, the patient will have less need to employ secondary defenses arising from anxiety, guilt, shame, or fear. As the patient regresses the staff takes increasing responsibility for his care. Part of this responsibility is to recognize when a patient is ready to start on the return journey.

Specific treatment plans must be established to meet the varied needs of individual patients. These needs are so varied that it is impossible to describe any single approach as the ideal. The optimal treatment setting must provide a broad range of therapeutic modalities. It must have the capacity to adapt continuously to the changing requirements of the individual patient.

4

DISCHARGE FROM THE PSYCHIATRIC HOSPITAL

Adequate planning for a patient's discharge from a psychiatric hospital involves the recognition and application of the following principles:

1. Discharge planning should begin at the time of admission to the hospital and should be an integral part of the patient's treatment.
2. The patient, the patient's family, the hospital, and the patient's community should participate in the planning.
3. The transition should be gradual.

Discharge from a mental hospital is a complex experience for the patient. He is forced either to re-establish or to develop personal ties with other people. As a result of his illness and his hospitalization, his personal relationship with others may have been interrupted or even severed. Some patients, because of the nature of their illness, may never have had close personal ties prior to their hospitalization.

The hospital treatment is designed to cope with both the degree of the patient's disorganization of adaptive functioning and the amount of his regression. The greater the patient's regression, the greater may be the breach between the patient, his family, and his community. Just as the depth of regression affects the treatment program, so does it affect the planning for the re-alliance of the patient with his community. Both treatment and discharge planning are concerned with the nature of the patient's illness and with his experience of separation from family, friends, and community.

As these very problems are being treated within the hospital, there is a concurrent and beginning phase of transition from the hospital to the community. Frequently the patient's illness requires resolution not only by the patient but also by his family and his community. The illness that has been symptomatically expressed by the patient is frequently more than a reflection of an intrapsychic disturbance. It can both reflect and cause a disturbance in the equilibrium between the patient, his family, and his community.

The patient's readiness for discharge is signalled by changes in the patient and in his interactions with his family. However, the assessment of the change is difficult and often controversial. At times symptomatic change may mask serious, continuing underlying disturbance. On the other hand, it is not unusual for some patients to retain symptoms while simultaneously demonstrating an increased capacity for adaptation. Sometimes symptomatic improvement leading to premature discharge occurs before the continuing disturbance in the equilibrium of the individual and his family is fully resolved. This may occur, for example, in response to psychotropic drugs or during the course of therapeutic explorations. However, improvement may crumble again unless there has been more than symptomatic change both in the patient and in the original disharmony.

Not every hospital can treat all patients. Nowhere is this more evident than in the efforts that lead to discharge. A hospital may not have sufficient assets and facilities. For example, the small community hospital or the psychiatric ward of a general hospital cannot easily provide for vocational rehabilitation, education, or job training for children or adolescents, halfway houses, or foster homes. If a hospital is unable to provide adequately for the patient's treatment, transfer of the patient to another hospital, rather than premature discharge, is advisable.

Case Example

A woman in her late 20's, married at age 18, felt overwhelmed by the active demands of her two children upon her. She became increasingly resentful, complained of her husband's lack of support, and felt guilty when, in a fury, she beat the children. As she became guilty, depressed, and suicidal, she was admitted to the psychiatric service of a general hospital. While her husband had magical expectations for a rapid cure with drugs, it was apparent that more intensive psychiatric treatment and care were indicated. The psychiatric ward was not suitably equipped for this task and a transfer was arranged. The patient was then treated for a two-month period in another hospital with an intensive milieu program that included individual and group therapy. On her discharge arrangements were made for continuing psychotherapy on an outpatient basis.

In an effort to solve the long-standing problems of chronic hospitalization, the pendulum has now swung in the direction of rapid and premature discharges from the hospital. These discharges frequently occur before treatment is completed and prior to adequate preparation for the patient's return to his community. The enthusiasm for rapid discharge has influenced psychiatric care and may interfere with patient welfare, just as delayed discharge may similarly impede the patient's progress.

Many patients require continuing support from the hospital. Some can maintain themselves in the community with the aid of mental health professionals. Despite all therapeutic efforts that may be made, it should be recognized that some patients may never achieve full or even limited discharge from a hospital. Nonetheless, many of these patients do achieve an equilibrium within the hospital setting. Only the mental hospital can adequately cope with these problems, and our zeal to work in the community and return patients rapidly home should not lead us to neglect the chronically disabled.

It is particularly in marginal situations that the continuing influence of the hospital upon the general community may alter the balance favorably for the patient. Not all patients can leave a mental hospital. Many have fears about their capacity to survive in the community even though they can establish a creative and active role for themselves in the hospital. And their families also fear being overburdened.

Case Example

> A patient in his late 70's was admitted in a confused state following a mild stroke. After recovery from the acute phase of his vascular accident, it was observed that the patient had residual memory loss, difficulty with attention span, and a severe tremor. In planning for his return to the community, it was anticipated that someone would have to assume initiative in providing assistance with making day-to-day decisions, including basic personal care and social contacts. The hospital social worker explained the patient's limitations to the community family agency that then made arrangements for a visiting nurse. His niece and nephew found an apartment close to their home and also agreed to accompany the patient initially on his return visits to the hospital for follow-up care. Were it not for the fact that the hospital agreed to accept the patient back on visits and offered support to the relatives, their participation would not have been likely.

Hospital followup facilities, local social agencies, and the patient's private physician can be sources of support in the post-hospitalization period. These may include halfway houses, vocational rehabilitation, social clubs for patients, family agencies, foster care, and the like. Again the broad range of hospital and community facilities necessary for optimal patient care is apparent. The availability of these resources may lessen the opportunity or need for further or repeated regressions.

Both internal psychic conflicts and the stresses of the external environment must be altered so that a new and healthier equilibrium is established. It is often possible to return a patient home rapidly after symptomatic improvement has occurred but without real psychological change. The adolescent on medication who is no longer deluded or hallucinated may in no way be ready to cope with the return to the family environment in which his disorganization began. The disappearance of anxiety and depression in a mother with postpartum depression does not mean that the mother is ready and able to care for her infant and her family responsibilities.

When critical intrapsychic conflicts have been resolved, the patient is better able to cope with the outside world. However, those external factors that have been unduly stressful and that have contributed to a breakdown of the patient's defenses may still exist.

The assessment of the external stresses may best be done by the family physician and local social agencies whose visits to the home can produce essential data for the patient and the hospital staff. It is also possible to test new adaptations by introducing some of the stresses of the home into the hospital. Thus, a mother might strengthen her ability to care for her children through visiting them at home or having them visit her on the ward of the hospital for increasing periods of time and with gradually lessening hospital support. In other instances a homemaker may facilitate the transitions of discharge.

Sometimes the patient should not return directly to the stresses of home after leaving the hospital. This is often necessary for adolescents or young adults for whom other living arrangements are more therapeutic. They may enter into a "halfway" home situation or an independent living arrangement. Under these circumstances, it is especially important that the family lend its support and understanding in achieving a new equilibrium in the face of feelings of painful separation and loss.

Case Example

> A 16-year-old girl ran away from home in response to continuing family disturbance and agitation. The parents were repeatedly and frequently engaged in verbal battles, and the girl was severely and punitively restricted. She ran away without clothes or money and was "picked up" by an older man. When found by the police she was hysterical, refused to return home, and was temporarily hospitalized. In planning the girl's discharge, arrangements were made for her to live at some distance

from her family with family friends who had daughters her age and who were capable of providing a sympathetic but structured family and school setting. Referral was made to a local family agency who helped her resume her schooling and, following her graduation from high school, helped with job placement.

Discharge from a hospital involves the basic psychodynamic problems of disequilibrium, separation, and reintegration. Separation from the hospital is part of the process of recovery. It touches upon fundamental aspects of character structure and may reawaken many of the conflicts that initially led to hospitalization. The principles outlined above stress that separation should be gradual rather than abrupt and that changes in both the patient and his environment may be necessary to foster human growth.

We have discussed the particular problems associated with discharge from the hospital. Certain of these require for optimal management a broad range of special personnel and facilities. It is difficult to provide these in the small psychiatric unit. There is also the problem of the marginally or chronically disabled patient —the hard core of the mentally ill. These are easy to forget, difficult to work with, and win few votes. Nonetheless, they are people, and our growing interest in the community should not lead us to overlook their tragedy or our ignorance of ways to alleviate it. We have emphasized the necessity for altering both the patient's ways of coping with his life stresses and the strength of the stress to which he is subject. If nothing is changed in this situation—if the patient's symptoms have been suppressed to achieve an early discharge—the hospitalization has been useless for the patient.

5

CURRENT CONTROVERSIES AND FUTURE DIRECTIONS

We have written about a current dilemma in psychiatry. A complex "movement" has evolved that in its most extreme form is represented by three slogans regarding psychiatric hospitals: "Keep patients out of hospitals"; "Use the psychiatric ward of a general hospital rather than a specialized psychiatric hospital"; and "The only good psychiatry is community psychiatry."

We are critical of this movement away from the psychiatric hospital. Our criticism is based on both theoretical and clinical considerations. With regard to *theory,* the slogans are not sufficiently related to a concept of individual personality development and personality breakdown or to the specialized needs of the patient. The *clinical* result of uncritical acceptance of these slogans leads to diagnostic and treatment errors. Readmission rates are increasing in ways that are antitherapeutic. A large number of semifunctioning individuals are immobilized through misuse of medications.

People cannot be treated by slogans or concepts. Hospital psychiatry or community psychiatry taken as an abstraction cannot treat or cure people. People treat people. Patients' emotional conflicts are altered as the result of human interactions. Such interactions may occur in many different settings: the home, the school, the church, the community recreation center, the physician's office, the general hospital, *or* the psychiatric hospital. We are in favor of diversifying and increasing the locales where therapeutic interactions may occur, but we object to those trends that attempt to exclude the psychiatric hospital from the possible therapeutic locales.

The psychiatric controversy and dilemma central to this report involve but a few basic issues, but they are significant and have many ramifications for patient care. The first issue that has been implied but not detailed in this report involves fundamental concepts about psychiatric illness. Both the professionals and the public are sharply divided in their perspectives toward psychiatric problems and their treatment, despite frequent lip service to a holistic concept of mental health and mental illness.

One extreme position is represented by those who regard psychiatric disorders as the result of organic dysfunctions. With such a theory of etiology the locale of treatment is significant only to the extent that it provides access to the prompt and efficient application of somatic remedies. Another extreme position is represented by those who believe that only current social forces are of significance in the etiology and the treatment of mental illness. Such a view assumes that any setting can be molded to meet the needs of all patients. A third extreme position narrowly regards pathological regression, anxiety, depression, and aggression as symptoms resulting entirely from intrapsychic conflict; it also ignores the social and biological factors. Such a position assumes that therapeutic change takes place in a social and biological vacuum. We advocate an approach that encompasses biological, social, and intrapsychic factors in a concept of mental health and the etiology of mental illness.

Symptoms of mental illness emerge when an individual's defenses cannot cope with the quantity or quality of his current life stresses, whether the origin of the stresses be primarily intrapsychic, organic, or determined by the patient's environment. The nature of the symptoms reflects the current level of personality functioning and/or underlying defects in personality development. The patient's symptoms already represent his effort to return to a more stable level of adjustment. With this concept of symptom formation mental health professionals can decide on the appropriate means for treating the individual patient. The complexity of the human problems encountered in clinical practice requires diversified therapeutic approaches.

A second issue in the present controversy about psychiatric hospitals has to do with the psychiatric units in general hospitals. These units were created for good reasons. The traditional private or public mental hospital was often psychologically and geographically distant. These distances often caused a separation of the patient from his home-base and from his home-doctor that was antitherapeutic. The long-term orientation of many traditional psychiatric hospitals frequently encouraged regression because of social isolation. The psychiatric units of general hospitals were initially designed to correct the above defects through immediate, local, and short-term treatment of psychiatric patients.

There are, however, major limitations in the goals that can be achieved by the general hospital psychiatric unit and major difficulties in the implementation of these goals. The units can provide only a limited spectrum of care. With their necessary requirement of short-term hospitalization, they offer chiefly diagnostic services and therapeutic techniques oriented toward rapid symptom remission and discharge. They cannot meet the need of many patients for a wider range of therapeutic care and more extended hospitalization.

Frequently the psychiatric unit is regarded as a strange and alien body within the general hospital. There are pressures to structure the psychiatric ward in the pattern of the medical ward. The staff may not be able to provide the occupational, recreational, and rehabilitative activities needed by patients. Disturbing behavior is more difficult to tolerate and manage, and it is more likely to be controlled by social pressure or by excessive medication. The nursing personnel on these units are frequently viewed by their hospital supervisors and peers as a "deviant" group. If there are personnel shortages, inadequately prepared nonpsychiatric personnel may be pressed into service.

In some cases, general hospital psychiatric units function as small psychiatric hospitals and perform most or all of the functions we have described above. This is most likely to occur when the psychiatric unit has a good deal of administrative autonomy —when it has a well-trained staff and the freedom to develop its own program. More often, however, the psychiatric unit operates simply as an adjunct to the medical and surgical services and is highly constrained by the policies and attitudes of the general hospital. In these cases it is very difficult to establish an effective therapeutic program.

A third issue facing psychiatry is the increasing expectation and demand for clinical service. The community mental health movement has attempted the laudable goal of rectifying class discrimination in psychiatric treatment. In moving toward this goal it is difficult to avoid making promises that exceed our manpower and our capacity for effective action. Legislators often fund programs on the basis of promises to treat more people for a cost lower than that of hospital treatment. Even if the prediction that community mental health centers will save money in the long run proves to be true, the pressure involved in the creation of new community mental health centers will adversely affect those patients who require hospital care. A new form of opprobrium has begun to be attached to psychiatric hospitalization that is not based upon clinical evidence or upon social psychiatric research. We are deeply concerned that demeaning the importance of psychiatric hospitals may result in the loss of public support for both psychiatric hospitals and community mental health centers.

*　*　*

This report was written to call attention to a major dilemma facing American psychiatry. We are clinicians concerned with the problems of people. We believe that psychiatric hospitals serve a unique function for many patients. The extension of mental health services from hospital and clinic into the community is progressive, and we support this long-overdue direction in psychiatry. But we protest against the view that psychiatric hospitalization is a sign of failure of alternate methods of therapeutic care.

This report has identified the unique functions of psychiatric hospitalization. These functions can complement the community mental health programs and thus meet the needs of the troubled people to whom this report is dedicated.

Acknowledgments

The program of the Group for the Advancement of Psychiatry, a non-profit, tax-exempt organization, is made possible largely through the voluntary contributions and efforts of its members. For their financial assistance during the past fiscal year, in helping it to fulfill its aims, GAP is grateful to the following foundations and organizations:

Sponsors

    CIBA CORPORATION
    THE DIVISION FUND
    MAURICE FALK MEDICAL FUND
    THE GRANT FOUNDATION
    THE HOFFMANN-LaROCHE FOUNDATION
    ITTLESON FAMILY FOUNDATION
    PARKE, DAVIS & COMPANY
    SANDOZ PHARMACEUTICALS
    SQUIBB INSTITUTE FOR MEDICAL RESEARCH
    SMITH KLINE & FRENCH FOUNDATION
    THE UPJOHN COMPANY
    WALLACE PHARMACEUTICALS

Donors

    GRALNICK FOUNDATION
    MORRIS AND SOPHIE KARDON FOUNDATION

Publications of the
Group for the Advancement of Psychiatry

Because readers of this publication may not be aware of previously published GAP titles, a selected listing is given below:

Number	Title	Price
46	ADMINISTRATION OF THE PUBLIC PSYCHIATRIC HOSPITAL—July 1960	$1.00
51	TOWARD THERAPEUTIC CARE: A GUIDE FOR THOSE WHO WORK WITH THE MENTALLY ILL—Oct. 1961	2.50
55	PUBLIC RELATIONS: A RESPONSIBILITY OF THE MENTAL HOSPITAL ADMINISTRATOR—April 1963	.75
58	MEDICAL PRACTICE AND PSYCHIATRY: THE IMPACT OF CHANGING DEMANDS—Oct. 1964	.75
*S-10	URBAN AMERICA AND THE PLANNING OF MENTAL HEALTH SERVICES—Nov. 1964	2.00
61	LAWS GOVERNING HOSPITALIZATION OF THE MENTALLY ILL—May 1966	.50
64	EDUCATION FOR COMMUNITY PSYCHIATRY—March 1967	1.00
69	THE DIMENSIONS OF COMMUNITY PSYCHIATRY—March 1968	1.00
70	THE NONPSYCHOTIC ALCOHOLIC PATIENT AND THE MENTAL HOSPITAL (A Position Statement)—Oct. 1968	.25

S refers to Symposium.

Orders amounting to less than $3.00 must be accompanied by remittance. All prices are subject to change without notice.

GAP publications may be ordered on a subscription basis. The current subscription cycle comprising the Volume 7 Series covers the period from July 1, 1968 to June 30, 1971. The subscription fee is $12.00 U.S.A. and $13.00 Canadian and other foreign, payable in U.S. currency.

Bound volumes of GAP publications issued since 1947 are also available. They include GAP titles no longer in print that are unavailable in any other form.

Please send your order and remittance to: Publications Office, Group for the Advancement of Psychiatry, 419 Park Avenue South, New York, New York 10016.

This publication was produced for the Group for the Advancement of Psychiatry by the Mental Health Materials Center, Inc., New York.